The Little Hormone
That Can

The Little Hormone That Can

NORMA JEANNE CERESIA

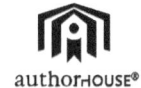

authorHOUSE®

AuthorHouse™
1663 Liberty Drive
Bloomington, IN 47403
www.authorhouse.com
Phone: 1-800-839-8640

njc@tan2lose.com
tan2lose.com

First published by AuthorHouse   11/15/2011

ISBN: 978-1-4678-5359-0 (sc)
ISBN: 978-1-4678-5358-3 (hc)
ISBN: 978-1-4678-5357-6 (ebk)

Library of Congress Control Number: 2011919613

Printed in the United States of America

Acknowledgments

Many thanks to my family for their support and belief in my ideas; to my doctors, who supported and encouraged my weight loss efforts; and to Lauren Studios in Albany, New York, for searching their archives for my "before" pictures and the wonderful cover photos.

Contents

Foreword by Sharon Alger-Mayer MD, Daniel Esper, MD, FACC, FSCAI, and Marie Schongar, MS, FNP-C, BC—ADM, CDE

Foreword

Norma has made an incredible wellness journey over the past five years and has improved her health and vitality. Her struggle began years earlier, when despite normal body weight throughout childhood, she noticed her weight increasing in her early twenties, despite no changes in her diet or activity patterns. She was diagnosed with hypothyroidism and started on thyroid hormones, but continued to gain weight, reaching a top weight of 248 pounds in 2004. She attempted numerous diet plans, and would successfully drop 10-15 pounds but would rapidly regain the weight.

At the time of her initial evaluation in July 2006 she was at high risk for heart disease due to elevated cholesterol and metabolic syndrome. In addition she struggled with severe fatigue and D deficiency.

Over the past five years Norma has lost nearly seventy pounds, dropping from a weight of 248 to 166 pounds. Her blood sugar levels have normalized. She reports major improvement in her energy level and quality of life. She is exercising on a regular basis. We applaud her efforts on her journey toward health and wellness.

Sharon Alger-Mayer, MD
Associate Professor of Medicine
Albany Medical College

*   *   *

Mrs. Ceresia has done well from a cardiovascular health maintenance perspective when she has included careful, gradual weight reduction with appropriate activity levels. Her personal sense of "being healthy" has improved significantly while following such a program. Not only has her blood pressure and lipid management been better, but she has been able to reduce her medication requirements as we work toward well established guidelines set forth by the American College of Cardiology/American Heart Association. For the past twelve years she has shown the benefits of an aerobic based activity program with careful weight reduction in her daily routine.

Daniel Esper, MD FACC, FSCAI

Although Norma is not one of my patients, I have seen in her the struggles of living with being overweight and having diabetes that many of my own patients have to cope with every day. Following a diet, exercising, testing blood sugars and taking daily medications to get blood sugars under great control becomes a "job" in itself for many of my patients. Norma has worked so hard over the years to lose weight by trying many different traditional diet methods, but her newest adventure has finally paid off. I could see that her stamina had improved for even just walking. Norma describes her journey eloquently in this book. This unique approach to combating obesity and diabetes can help you to make major lifestyle changes to enjoy a healthier, happier life and prevent the complications from diabetes.

Marie Schongar, MS, FNP-C, BC—ADM, CDE
Director of Diabetes Education Program
Capital Care
Schenectady, NY

Introduction

If you are frustrated with your weight loss efforts, this is the book for you. If you have tried all different types of weight loss programs and either couldn't lose the weight that you wanted to or lost it but gained it all back again, then this is the book for you. These scenarios were mine before I realized that I needed a new approach. I was desperate; it seemed my body wasn't obeying all the rules. I went to doctor after doctor, why didn't I fit the mold? It looked like I wasn't even trying or I was making excuses for overeating. The exact opposite was true. It was so frustrating and embarrassing. I knew that if I were to be successful, I had to look for the answers myself, so I took a scientific approach.

This book is about an entirely different approach to weight loss. It uses current scientific research, common sense, logic, reason, and a critically important hormone, melanocyte stimulating hormone (MSH), that you already have and will learn how to very easily control to help you create your own, personalized system for your weight loss journey. You will design a system just for you. It will be different from anyone else's, so it will be easier for you to use and much more efficient for reaching your weight loss goal. You will use lots of data that you will collect and learn how to analyze and manipulate to reach your goal weight.

On my weight loss journey, I discovered the usefulness of MSH, which has totally transformed my life and helped me lose weight quickly, efficiently, and permanently. I will show you how to make it work for you, and I will back it up with scientific principles to support my claims. I will give you information so you can make your own decisions based on fact and not on what other people may think will be helpful. However well-intentioned others are, you are the only one who can develop a program that will be successful for you. While making decisions for yourself, your tools for this experience will be your powers of observation. You will take command of your body by getting to know how it functions.

There are almost seven billion people in this world and we all have the human elements in common. We eat, sleep, breathe and have emotions and intellect. This is all determined by a molecule called DNA. This encodes all of the features of our being. As sure as we all are similar, we are also very different. So different that we use our DNA to distinguish between each individual with such accuracy that we can convict a person of a crime based on just one sample of DNA and how it differs from all others.

So then why, when it comes to making decisions for our very unique selves, do we rely on information that is based on the masses of humanity? Do we really expect our bodies to react in the same manner as everyone else's? Do you have the same allergies as everyone you know? Is your eyesight the same? No, of course not! Why then, should we lump ourselves into the same group "human" and assume that we all will lose weight on the same weight loss program?

Accepting the fact that we are all different is the key to this weight-loss adventure. The first piece of evidence that this is true is something that you have already observed. You know people that can consume large amounts of food and remain excruciatingly thin. You also know people who consume very little and yet remain overweight and are seemingly helpless to control it. This is a very discouraging scenario, I see it every day and I experienced it myself for far too many years. I used to blame it on my DNA to try to console myself. I just assumed that my family must have the "fat gene." I have frustrated myself to tears trying to do what was working for "everyone else." It didn't work for me. No surprise, I am not the same as "everyone." I am me, and I realized that I had to learn about my own body and how it functions before I could expect weight loss success.

You will learn how to experiment to find out how your body works. You will discover what data to analyze and how to use reason to get answers for yourself. You will begin to have the confidence to seek alternatives, answers, and techniques that are unique to you, that work for you, and that will empower and give you the confidence necessary to solve your own problems. Rejoice that you are a unique individual, and enjoy this journey of discovery.

I will share my personal adventure and how a unique set of circumstances has led me to discover this technique and the science behind it. Using the techniques in this book, you will create a program specifically for you, and your experience will be successful and rewarding.

CHAPTER ONE

We Are Doing it All Wrong

Nowhere is it more important to take an objective look at how we view something than with obesity. For all the hype and all the research, we still haven't found out how to solve the problem. Actually, the answer is all around us and we keep hiding from "it," which is actually the problem. "The answer" is the sun. Think about it: obesity rates have skyrocketed in all age groups, even in our young children. Osteoporosis is a menace for older people and has crippling effects. Type 2 diabetes and metabolic syndrome are looming at our door.

We can detect, diagnose, and use Band-Aid treatments for these health issues, but identifying the causes and prevention remain elusive. To solve the problem, we must look at ourselves as an integral part of our environment. We influence our environment and it influences us. To almost completely block a major environmental factor out of our lives is most definitely going to have a dramatic effect on our well-being. By this I mean hiding from the rays of the sun.

Humans have evolved on earth under the rays of the sun for millions of years. We are dependent on the sun to provide heat, food, daylight, and oxygen, yet we ignore the fact that there are health benefits that we derive from exposure. It's true that people can get melanoma from the sun, but don't ignore the fact that some melanomas occur where the sun does not usually shine, such as the bottoms of the feet, in between toes, and in armpits.

Exposure to the sun causes humans to produce MSH, melanocyte stimulating hormone. (1)This is the hormone that causes us to tan. It protects us, and like most other hormones, performs other functions as well.

If we view humans as creatures that have evolved over time, we can understand where and how these functions assist in our survival. We consume calories for energy when they are available, use what we need at the moment, and store the rest in different forms, one of which is fat, for later use when food is less available. Therefore, there must be a signal for us to store excess calories as well as a signal that tells us to utilize our fat stores for energy. Melanocyte stimulating hormone serves as the signal that alerts the body that there is fat available to utilize.

Up until now we have limited our understanding of fat utilization to creating a caloric deficit by dieting and utilizing energy by exercising. In a perfect world, that makes sense. But what if your body's signal is turned off? What if your body is crying for calories and it doesn't get the signal that there is available fat to use? The result is that your body's survival instinct activates. You get hungry, and if you are dieting and do not act on that signal, you get very hungry, even ravenous, and you may begin to tremble as a result of lowered blood sugar levels. This is a basic survival instinct, and when in this condition it is almost impossible to avoid eating. Even worse is that now you need calories that can be quickly digested and enter into your bloodstream fast. The choice is carbohydrates.

It is almost guaranteed that you will consume far more calories than you actually need, and so you will store the excess as fat. It is virtually impossible to eat exactly the number of calories that your body needs at each moment, twenty-four hours a day, and so with this lack of a fat-burning signal to your body, you are now on the fast track to weight gain, metabolic syndrome, and if you continue on this path, to type 2 diabetes.

I wrote this book to teach you how to provide for your metabolic needs so you can function properly. The sun is an integral part of this process because it causes your body to produce melanocyte stimulating hormone. Weight loss can be achieved by maintaining your metabolism so it can burn the calories you need and also enabling your body to produce the hormones that drive your signaling system. This way you will burn the available calories stored in your fat reserves instead of causing you to go into the starvation mode, which will make you consume an overabundance of calories which will in turn be stored as fat.

This is an all too familiar scenario. You have an important social engagement, so you restrict your calories so you can fit into those new clothes. You take off a few pounds, which all too often is mostly water weight and intestinal contents. You can control yourself until after the event, at which time you go into starvation mode. This forces you to consume so many calories that you end up back where you started or worse. This can be a never ending scenario. I will teach you how to get off of this not-so-merry go round.

I will share my voyage of discovery including the unique situations that made me aware of the process happening in my own body. I will dismiss current myths of weight loss. You will learn how to choose a doctor who is willing to listen to you (there are many that won't). You will decide what factors you need to track to accumulate the information you will use to make successful weight loss decisions. Each person is a unique individual, so each person should have his or her own unique program. This will enable you to care for your metabolism and provide everything it needs to function well. You will also learn about the systems of the human body. There is a chapter on tricks and techniques of weight loss, and I describe physiological conditions that you probably already encounter and teach you how to deal with them.

Currently, obesity is viewed as an epidemic. All you have to do is look around. Everywhere I go I see people dealing with the very severe effects of obesity, which not only impacts their health, but limits their everyday mobility. My concern is that our children are going to be dealing with these problems for a lifetime. As you apply the principles in this book to your own health and diet issues, do not forget that children are being affected by obesity at an alarming rate. This is happening for the same reasons that obesity is happening to adults.

When our children play indoors, they do not get the benefits of minimal sun exposure.

They become hungrier and more sedentary, which is exacerbated by low levels of MSH, and thus the cycle repeats itself, bringing us to the crisis stage that we have now in this country.

Have a serious conversation with your children's pediatrician about limited sun exposure; follow the doctor's instructions on how to have your children go outside for a short time on a limited schedule. Let them get a small amount of sun for a few minutes and then apply photoprotection. Again, follow your doctor's guidelines. Your children will gradually become more active and less hungry as their levels of MSH increase. Make sure you provide healthy snacks and plenty of liquids. Participate with them in fun activities like hiking, swimming, bike riding, or playing ball. Whatever interests them and keeps the whole family moving together is a good thing. Adopt your new healthier lifestyle and enjoy sharing with each other. Chart your child's progress and let them participate in the process so it becomes a habit that they will continue on their own later on. You will be teaching them healthy habits that will last a lifetime.

As you read this book, make a decision that this is a new day and a better way to accomplish your goals, reduce your stress, and get lasting results utilizing the functions that your body already has in place.

CHAPTER TWO

Voyage of Discovery

My personal story will show how I came to the information that eventually changed my life. Through a very unique set of circumstances I was thrust into the position of making this monumental discovery.

As a child I was naturally thin. It didn't take much effort. I ate what I wanted, which was, of course, candy. I had energy to burn and a slim, tall frame. Even so, I was extremely focused on my body and my weight. I think it was because both of my parents were overweight and I saw how they struggled. At that young age I knew that I was looking at my future, so I became very careful. My parents were on board also because they didn't want me to have to deal with obesity. My mother helped by giving me goals to achieve. The most helpful goal that I remember was to remain under one hundred pounds until my thirteenth birthday, which was about ten months away. If I made the goal, I would get money for a new outfit. No specific diet or rules had to be followed; that was up to me. Simple, yet this kept me on track for ten months. I learned to control my diet, and I achieved my goal. It was important to me to monitor my weight on a daily basis. Support of family and friends was very important and helped in my success. I can actually remember what I weighed at certain points in my life, even when I was thin.

It is important to mention here that we lived in Connecticut, a state where it was sunny, though not always hot, most of the time. We spent a lot of time at the beach during the summer months. Then I went to college in an area that was cloudy and overcast most of the time. It didn't matter much to me; I studied most of the time and therefore wasn't outside anyway.

College years are typically harder for weight control. Everyone talks about the freshman fifteen. Usually people attribute it to all the time spent studying and a change in available food choices. I assumed it would come off during the summer, and it usually did. However, during this period I gradually had to restrict my calories more and more, I did so and graduated tall and thin.

Then I became employed and I had to deal with another change in life and routine. I lived in the same geographic area as the college that I attended. This time I found that it was not only more difficult to lose weight but much easier to gain weight. Feeling frustrated and becoming fearful that I was losing control, I went to a doctor. It was a great advantage to have observed myself over the years. I could accurately describe my problem. He went right for the thyroid and he was correct. I had Hashimoto's disease. My own body was producing antibodies that were destroying my thyroid. The thyroid produces hormones that control metabolism. That was why I was gaining weight. However, he said that taking a little hormone pill every day would replace what I didn't make anymore and that things would be back in balance.

Things were never the same. The weight went on and it didn't come off. That isn't to say that it didn't fluctuate, a celebration would come along and I would gain a pound, so I would restrict my calories and lose the pound. The weight would come back so much more quickly than before, and it would become a permanent resident. Now I know that this happened because the weight I lost wasn't fat. It was probably a combination of water and bowel contents from my dieting efforts. Looking back I can say that this is what was happening but at the time as my weight fluctuated it wasn't that obvious. On a good day I retained less fluid, so I lost a little weight. I would declare victory, only to have those nasty pounds creep back on. This was a sure sign of an internal signaling problem. The best way to describe it is a person can try to eat correctly for a day and fat would not build up or be lost. However, on a long term basis I could not maintain this balancing act.

On those occasional special days, such as Thanksgiving or Christmas, when typical people overindulge, the next day they adjust their caloric intake for a few days and the extra weight comes off. In my case I would lose water weight and the fat would still be there after I had erroneously declared victory. Whenever

I ate too much, the excess would be stored as fat, but when I restricted my calories I didn't lose the fat. With this scenario you can see that over time, even being as careful as you can, the weight is going to gradually build up. You can also see that it was a very confusing situation for me, being able to take off some weight but never as much as I gained. Each time this happened the scale kept creeping up.

I got married, and with each pregnancy came more pounds. All of these scenarios are easily accounted for—college, pregnancy, thyroid disease. I gradually found myself at 248 pounds, unbelievable, how could this be? I went from in control to being helpless.

Then I looked at my children. They were beginning to have the same weight problem that I was struggling with. My weight problem was one thing, but my children were a different story. I became obsessed—was I creating this? There is nothing more motivating than dealing with a problem that affects your own children. I had to figure this out.

I tried every diet known to man. I got packaged meals once a week. I didn't lose weight, and they had the nerve to tell me that I was wasting my time if I was going to cheat! I wasn't cheating; I just wasn't losing! I went to weekly diet meetings and joined aerobic dance classes, but nothing worked for me.

Finally, with the encouragement of his doctor, my twenty-one year old son and I started the Atkins Diet. Protein was king, and the more we ate the more we lost. It was great. After six weeks I had lost sixteen pounds, and my son was even more successful. We kept going, comparing victories, and he continued to have them, but I did not. Sixteen was it. I still had eighty to go, so for the next six months I kept the faith and followed the diet to the letter. My son's weight was plummeting down, and I was watching from the sidelines.

One of the great advantages of Atkins is that you can test for ketones and actually see if the diet affects your metabolism to help you lose weight. My son thought this was great; his test strip was deep purple, and mine was light pink. I did the ramped-up version of the diet to jump start my losses, and still nothing. No matter what I did, my body would not go into ketosis. When ketones are detected in your urine, it is proof that your body is burning fat. My son was; I wasn't. He lost sixty five pounds and I lost sixteen and I suspect that it was sixteen pounds of muscle and water not fat!

For the first time, I had inadvertently proven that people are different. Not all diets work for everybody. Now what? My fat wouldn't come off with a blow torch. I kept looking for an answer. Of course, I could still blame it on my thyroid, but my hormones were in balance. Then one day I was watching TV and saw a news piece about a new discovery from researchers at the Eleanor Roosevelt Institute at the University of Colorado. They showed obese mice that lacked the gene that produces MSH and when the mice were administered MSH they lost weight.

Being at the end of my frazzled rope, I called the two scientists to ask about the compound. I found out that it was many years and much experimentation away from human use. All I could do was wait. At a dead end and at the end of my wits, I conceded. No doctor, no scientist, no drug, nothing could help me at this point. Thank goodness that my son seemed to be successful on his diet.

My husband and I decided to take a road trip down south. Before we left I had an appointment with my general practitioner, who was patient with me and considered all I had to say. He said he would try a test for adrenal function, which involved an injection. I got it and left for vacation.

If you have ever been on a road trip, you know that it is sit and ride, stop to eat, and then keep on riding. This amount of inactivity is not exactly conducive to weight loss. But that first night as I lay in bed, I felt something I hadn't felt in years. When I had lost weight in my younger years, I had always felt emptiness in my stomach at night, almost like a gentle vacuum. I call this sensation, "feeling the burn." I told my husband about it and then went to sleep.

I haven't mentioned that my husband has always been in control of his weight, thin and in shape. While we were traveling, we ate basically the same things. When we got home, I had lost five pounds, and he was still the same weight. Wait a minute—something had just happened here. It had to have been caused by the injection of adrenocorticotropic hormone (ACTH) I got for the test. I now had undeniable results, cause and effect. I started to read about ACTH and MSH. In my research I discovered that the first thirteen amino acids of the ACTH and MSH molecules are exactly the same. This meant they could have similar effects, and I had inadvertently proven that they did. However, there was no way to get MSH, and ACTH is very powerful and not proven for nor prescribed for losing weight. I was so close and yet so far away.

I made an appointment with an endocrinologist, who did many tests including monitoring my thyroid and blood glucose levels. She found that I had type 2 diabetes and said that if I didn't take action now and lose the excess weight, I would likely have to deal with full-blown diabetes and all of the associated problems. I was only fifty-one, and I was on the verge of a debilitating illness. I would have done anything to lose weight, but I had no way to deal with my particular metabolic situation. I told her my story, and she referred me to her associate, Sharon Alger-Mayer, MD, who specializes in nutrition.

That was my lucky day! She listened intently to my story and said I could have my MSH levels tested. They were so low they couldn't be read with any accuracy. At that point I threw caution to the wind. I knew sun exposure is thought to be bad, but I couldn't help myself. I spent as much time outside as possible, at the beach, walking—you name it and I was out under the sun enjoying it.

I devised my own plan of calorie restriction, movement, and an attempt to stimulate my natural MSH levels. The pounds slowly started to come off, dieting was surely part of it, but it was working; this time my efforts were being rewarded. As I lost weight, I developed a tracking system. I wanted to know exactly what was working so I could keep doing it. I have lost eighty pounds so far, and I am still losing. I still have and always will have type 2 diabetes, but it is under the best control ever. I feel great and look better than I have in years. I don't want to keep these techniques a secret. I don't want people to waste their time and money on diets that won't work and will make them discouraged. I have created a plan that has increased my MSH levels, lowered my blood sugar levels, and enabled me to lose the excess weight. I have also created an information collection system for you to use so you can analyze your own data and follow a weight loss program that you have specifically designed for yourself.

Being successful at weight loss is exhilarating. As your efforts are rewarded, your resolve will increase; success is just around the corner. It's a new day—let's enjoy it!

CHAPTER THREE

Myths

Weight is a really personal thing; you might discuss it with others or you might not. One thing I can guarantee is that you fall prey to the supermarket magazines and television ads—you know, the ones that have the miracle cure for obesity. "You can lose 10, 20, 30 pounds before (insert the next holiday here)." I admit I do look at the pictures on the cover, but I don't waste my money . . . anymore. I asked myself, "If these diets had a shred of evidence that they worked, then why do they change every week?" And those pictures! A woman who lost eighty-plus pounds in a bikini? You really have to let go of the tendency to believe what you see, as pictures can be altered to make you believe in something that isn't true. That doesn't bother me, but the effect it can have on a person does. It gives people an unrealistic goal, and then they may get discouraged and give up when a realistic goal is actually attainable and desirable. Some of those diets may work for a little while, but they won't help you achieve lasting weight loss. What you lose won't be all stored fat, and eventually the weight will come back—and then some. This can be very devastating.

Let's get rid of the myths, they are holding you back., let them go!

Myth #1. Don't Weight Yourself Every Day.

Wrong! Weigh yourself morning, noon, and night if you want. The more information you gather, the better. All I suggest is that you keep meticulous records (I will provide you with a system later). All along this journey you are going to track, analyze, and adjust your techniques. As you learn more about your body and the way it works, the more valuable this data will become. I don't want you to spend months adjusting your program only to find out later on that you should have tracked additional data. The more data you collect, the better.

Myth #2. Drink Eight 8-Ounce Glasses of Water Every Day

Does everyone on the planet run the same marathon every day? This myth has been around far too long. The fact is, your body is made up of millions of chemical reactions; some put molecules together and some take them apart. This is called your metabolism. Metabolism is your friend if you know how to use it. Do you want to dilute your system to the point that the molecules cannot find each other fast enough? Would that not slow down your metabolic rate? People have died from consuming too much water. Your body has an entire system devoted to balancing the amount of water in your body. Why? Because it is just that important! Hormones will tell your kidneys to either save water or excrete the excess. There is a delicate balance here, so don't mess with it.

Myth #3. If You Wait Until You Feel Thirsty, it's Too Late!

Well, that's pretty grim. The fact is, we have evolved over millions and millions of years. We are the products of the genes that help us to survive in our world, a finely tuned instrument that contains information that gives us the survival advantage, and with survival comes reproduction. Our offspring will carry that survival code. If we didn't have that, we wouldn't be here. If our bodies didn't tell us when we are thirsty until it is too late, then we wouldn't have survived these millions and millions of years.

You must, and I emphasize must, learn to trust your body. It knows how to function. Does it need help once in a while? Of course it does. But in a normal situation and on a daily basis, no. Now, if you are running a marathon or working in the hot sun, always take in extra water. Hydration is important; drowning in your own fluids or stressing out your excretory system is not.

Myth #4. The Same Techniques and Procedures of Weight Loss Will Work for Everyone

As sure as we all are different there are going to be different techniques that work best for each individual. We have to use all the tools at our disposal to zero in on what techniques work best for us as unique individuals. If you want to help others, you must teach them the techniques of self-discovery and encourage them to develop their own plan.

Myth #5. Exercise Increases Your Metabolic Rate

I agree with this statement to a point, but I believe the increase is temporary and therefore the weight loss benefit is minimal. Of course it is beneficial to move yourself around and get your blood moving. It does take calories to move around, and it is good for your heart, blood vessels, mood, etc. You will feel more in control of your weight loss experience. People who are larger have a difficult time raising their level of activity. If done incorrectly, it will stress your cardiac, respiratory, excretory, and musculoskeletal systems. You must introduce movement slowly so as not to stress your body or actually make yourself hungry. Do not fall prey to the notion that you can exercise off extra calories that you have already consumed. A very important point is that **an exercise program is not a diet program.** The first step in your weight loss journey is to lose weight and to learn how to eat. The worst thing you can do is try to add exercise at the same time.

Make this journey one step at a time. Get the eating/dieting under control and learn what works best for you. When you are confident and starting to be successful and comfortable with your program, then consider adding another variable such as a modest "movement program". Your body will tell you when you are ready to increase the level of intensity. When you feel more energized, adjust your activities accordingly. Do not stress yourself or push to the point of exhaustion or injury. That would only be counterproductive.

Myth #6. Lose Weight by Limiting Your Intake to One or Two Food Groups

I enjoyed the Atkins diet—I could stay on it, food was easy to prepare, and it was delicious. I actually lost weight eating wings and bleu cheese. As I mentioned, my son and I went on Atkins together, and it was a great experience. As a matter of fact, I would recommend dieting with a close friend or family member. You can share goals, frustrations, and recipes and support each other. Just don't lose sight of the fact that your body needs a balanced diet and each person is different. Our journeys were as different as night and day, but what we did have in common was that the weight we lost came right back, with additional weight. This made me afraid to diet, because I could end up even heavier than if I did nothing. Little did I know that my Atkins adventure would be the beginning of my big "ah ha" moment.

Myth #7. Dieting is Misery, Deprivation, Slow, Boring etc.

No it isn't, when you are doing it right it is fun, empowering, and invigorating, and you will feel a tremendous sense of accomplishment. Your clothes will fit better, you will look better, feel better, have more energy, and people will begin to notice and compliment you.

Myth #8. Avoid the Sun at All Costs

You have heard the dire warnings—the sun is bad, you will wrinkle prematurely, your skin will look like leather, you will need a face lift at forty, and worst of all, you will get melanoma. These myths can be true if you overdo your exposure. In this program, the sun exposure suggested is minimal, and there are significant disadvantages to avoiding the sun. Again, remember that we evolved over millions of years and for most of them there was no sunscreen. Our skin not only forms a protective barrier, but it also participates metabolically in our well-being. Your skin manufactures vitamin D when exposed to the sun. This vitamin is important in bone growth and maintenance; it promotes calcium absorption, and it helps to maintain a beneficial phosphate/calcium balance. Vitamin D is also integral to the proper functioning of your metabolism.(2)

The Shakes

Today, for the first time in a long time, I experienced "the shakes," my term for low blood sugar. Each person may experience this differently. I feel empty, nervous, shaky, and panicky. The desire for food is overwhelming, and I need it now! You should be familiar with how you feel when you experience low blood sugar and be prepared with juice, a piece of fruit, or a health bar, depending on what medications you may be on for blood sugar control and what your actual levels are, be sure to follow your doctor's instructions for blood sugar control.

First you need to understand what causes this situation. Our bodies must perform a balancing act. Most of us take in calories three times a day, but our bodies use calories constantly. We have evolved with an internal system to accommodate for this situation. The calories are digested and enter our bloodstream. The necessary energy from these calories is either used or stored as fat, and there is long-term storage and short-term storage. Short-term storage is in the liver where the calories are readily accessible, and long-term storage is located in fat deposits. This balancing act is a perfect design for survival; insulin that is produced by the pancreas facilitates blood sugar use by the body cells. When additional calories are needed, the body signals this and it responds by releasing energy stored in fat.(3) Everyone is happy!

The problem begins when there is either no signal or a faulty signal to the body to release the calories stored in fat. In short, your body doesn't "know" that there is fat available to use. No matter how calorie deficient you are, your body is not going to give up the stored fat; instead you will get weaker and start to shake. Eventually you will be unable to resist fast calories until your blood sugar levels rise and your body is fueled again.

This is why some diets have you graze or eat small portions several times a day to keep your metabolism humming along. You are trying to artificially keep your blood sugar consistent when your body should be doing that job by using your stored fat. You cannot possibly make give-and-take adjustments to your intake to exactly match your metabolic needs. You wouldn't have time for anything else. No matter how in tune you are with your body you cannot adjust your intake to your needs every minute of every day and night. Even if you could; it would just result in the maintenance of your current weight. Losing weight would be a whole different story.

This situation is exactly what happened to me. It didn't make any sense at first. I would go on a calorie restricted diet and lose a few pounds, and then the weight loss would stop and I would cause a low blood sugar situation, which in turn would eventually cause me to add calories.

What was really happening was deceptive because I would lose a few pounds of water weight and think that I had been successful at losing some fat, and then the process would stop for no known reason. Once

I realized that it wasn't fat that I had lost but water and other components, I knew I had to search for a different answer. The new question was "Why am I not losing fat when I diet?"

The key to this conundrum was my metabolism. There was something wrong, the message of low blood sugar was not getting through, and my body needed to know that it could access the fat stores. The messenger is MSH.(4) You are probably familiar with *melanocyte*; it sounds like *melanin,* which is the chemical that gives you a tan. Melanin is stored in melanocytes, which are the cells in your skin that cause you to tan. Many chemicals in our bodies perform more than one duty.

Sometimes we get creative and find several different uses for a household product. Take baking soda, for example. We use it in baking, for stain removal while doing laundry, as an odor absorbent in the refrigerator, and even as toothpaste. Your body is designed to be efficient also. In a healthy, well-functioning human being, everything is there for a reason and most likely for several reasons. In most cases, one structure or chemical has many jobs to do.

Your skeleton facilitates movement; without it your body would be like a bean bag chair. It also serves as a storage area for minerals such as calcium. Blood is made in its bone marrow, and your skeleton protects organs such as the brain, spinal cord, heart, and lungs.

Your hormones can also perform many jobs. Melanocyte stimulating hormone is made by your body. When you are exposed to the sun, it is known to stimulate the melanin-producing cells in your skin to produce a tan to protect you from the harmful rays of the sun. It is in trials currently to aid people who have total sun intolerance, a condition called Erythropoietic protoporphyria, which is when even a tiny flash of light produces severe and scarring burns in some people. MSH was found to be effective and well tolerated to treat this condition. The drugs used to treat people for esophageal cancer can cause light intolerance. In trials they were treated with MSH, which successfully reduced the problem with light intolerance(5).

As we are exposed to the sun, the skin responds by producing MSH, which stimulates melanin production and also serves as a messenger to your metabolism that there is fat stored that can be used for energy.

The current popular opinion is that the sun is bad for you. Look around you. Mothers are slathering their children with SPF 50+ and using long sleeves and hats. What is the current major health problem of children? Being overweight! Adults avoid the sun like the plague and what happens? Our society is grossly overweight and dealing with the corresponding health problems. So we are barraged by diet plans! All sorts of diets, shakes, protein, mail meals, frozen dinners, miracle juices, powdered drinks, magic elixirs, and on and on.

Sun avoidance is causing another deficiency, vitamin D, which we need for strong bones. (6) What epidemic are we currently facing? Osteoporosis! People are loading themselves up with calcium and taking vitamin D. All you have to do is observe the world around you and use your common sense. Are animals getting osteoporosis? Do you really think the sun is that bad for you? Did we evolve over millions of years on the face of this earth under the rays of the sun only to find out that it kills us? Or did our bodies evolve to use the sun and the rain and the air and plants and animals to thrive and survive? What is a more reasonable way to view the world?

Whenever you see or hear some extreme opinion, do not automatically believe it. Instead, use your ability to reason. Does this information really make sense? Make your own observations and draw your own conclusions. I want you to learn to collect your data, lots of it, and use it to come to your own conclusions. Remember, we are all the same, yet we are all different. Learn how your own body functions and reacts to the world around it and become proficient in guiding yourself in life based on your own scientific data.

You will set up a data collection system and learn how to use that information to make decisions for your own specific body and the situation that you live in.

CHAPTER FIVE

The Natural World

Whenever I have an idea, I always try to be sure that it makes sense and is realistic. Melanocyte stimulating hormone must be useful in a larger scope than just tanning and weight loss. It must have other, broader survival applications for it to be a part of the natural world.

Thinking about it for a while I realized that having high levels of MSH would be beneficial not only for using fat stores for energy, but having low levels of MSH would be useful for creating fat stores for use at a later time. Hibernating bears come to mind as a good example. They don't all of a sudden look around and decide they should begin packing on the pounds for winter. It is not a conscious decision on their part. It must be a natural instinct caused by a change in their internal signals. We eat when we are hungry, and so do the bears. When the days begin to become shorter, the amount of MSH that their bodies produce decreases. When MSH levels are low, it signals the body to become hungrier (what I call the shakes) so they become ravenous, eat more, and save the excess calories in their fat stores. Their behavior changes, and they feed to decrease their hunger and thus increase their fat stores. Having low MSH levels prevents the signal to the body to burn the fat stores, so they are inadvertently preparing themselves for the long winter.

We know that MSH levels are increased by the sun shining on the skin, but bears have fur, so their skin is not totally exposed to the sun. Research demonstrates that ultraviolet irradiation of the eyes increases the concentration of MSH in plasma.(7) So this information solves the mystery with the bears, but it also pertains to humans. We shield our eyes from the sun with sunglasses. This is another area where we are restricting the access of the rays of the sun. I am not telling you to go out and stare at the sun. Many people make a fashion statement with sunglasses, myself included. Now I wear them when I need them and not every moment that I am outside. Again, this is an opportunity for you to have a discussion with your doctor or ophthalmologist and get his or her recommendations for use of sunglasses.

So now this makes more sense on a larger scale. You can see the usefulness of the MSH levels being controlled by the amount of available sunlight. As in most cases, we have to understand what role MSH plays in nature to understand why this signaling is important in species survival, which is why it has been included in the evolutionary package. When its role is clearly understood, we can learn to control this mechanism and use it to our best advantage.

CHAPTER SIX

Metabolic Syndrome

Obesity is one of the risk factors for developing metabolic syndrome. This syndrome is actually diagnosed by the presence of at least three of the following conditions:

- **abdominal obesity:** described as a large waistline, over thirty-five inches for women and over forty inches for men o **high levels of fasting blood sugar:** indicates your carbohydrates are not being used efficiently by your cells; also known as insulin resistance.

o **low levels of HDL (high-density lipoprotein):** the good cholesterol that helps prevent damaging plaque buildup in your arteries

o **high blood pressure:** can damage arteries

o **high levels of triglycerides:** type of fat in the blood that can be very damaging to your blood vessels

o **elevated C-reactive protein:** also known as a pro-inflammatory state, which predisposes you to blood clots

o **elevated fibrinogen or plasminogen activator-1:** predisposing you to blood clots

Metabolic syndrome can lead to increased risk for stroke, heart disease, and diabetes (which carries with it the risks associated with diabetes, including circulatory problems and eye and kidney damage).(8)

All of these problems are extremely undesirable, and you should pursue the opportunity to reduce your risk of dealing with these conditions. In general, a healthier lifestyle will lower your risk factors. Lose weight, eat fewer fatty foods, reduce your blood sugar levels by eating a balanced diet including complex carbohydrates, increase your physical activity, quit smoking, and keep track of your body mass index. A body mass calculator can be found online, and you can enter different weights to see what you have to weigh to be considered normal. Using this information, you will be able to set goals for yourself.

Insulin resistance can also develop, which will affect your metabolism. Insulin is the hormone that controls your blood sugar levels and cell growth. If you have an unhealthy lifestyle, your cells can eventually become resistant to the effects of insulin, so your body needs more and more insulin to get the same result. If this downward spiral is not stopped, it can eventually lead to type 2 diabetes, which requires control by diet, oral or injectable medications, and/or additional insulin to maintain a healthy blood sugar level.

It is important to become informed about how the human body functions so you can make decisions concerning your dietary requirements. This will enable you to make use of your personal data and knowledge to make adjustments and decisions regarding your personalized diet program.

Human Body Facts

So far I have discussed some of the basic facts of weight loss. Now let's look at the entire human body—how it is built, why it reacts the way it does, and how you can use this knowledge to achieve your goals. Our bodies are a functioning unit the purpose of which is to maintain itself by reacting to changes in the external and internal environment. To this end there are systems that work together and are dependent on each other to help you to survive in your environment and to produce offspring.

The Senses (sight, smell, hearing, touch, and taste): Note that most of these senses are located in the head area. This is usually the first area we use to meet the outside world and where the information collected is processed and responses are formulated. The senses are our connection with the outside world.

The Integumentary System: Consists of the skin and components that cover the body. It protects us from damage and infection, regulates water loss, and controls body temperature. No matter the conditions outside the body, the internal conditions must be kept within narrow limits. When conditions are within these limits, we call this *homeostasis*.

Musculoskeletal System: Provides for movement, protection of internal organs, storage of minerals, and production of blood and its components.

Circulatory System: Transports oxygen, nutrients, waste products, and immune system components to the body. It carries wastes and water to be eliminated and nourishment for the body cells and components for the defense against disease.

Nervous System: Transports information from the senses to the brain and spinal cord for processing and carries the response to the muscles and organs.

Digestive System: Manages the intake of food, which is then digested into a usable form called nutrients, which are absorbed into the body and used for energy or stored. Food waste is not absorbed and passes through the digestive system to the rectum and anus, where it is eliminated.

Excretory System: This system is involved in maintaining water balance and removing metabolic wastes such as uric acid, urea, and excess salt.

Type 2 Diabetes

Type 2 or adult onset diabetes is a growing problem. More and more people are either dealing with this condition themselves, know someone who is dealing with it, or are caring for someone that has it. When I was diagnosed with type 2 diabetes, it really scared me. I knew what the usual outcome was—full-blown diabetes with the accompanying blood sugar testing, watching your diet, and an increased risk for heart disease, stroke, and circulation problems that could possibly lead to amputations or more medication by mouth or by injection.

I wanted no part of this scenario. My doctor said that I needed to lose weight, exercise, and watch my diet and blood sugar levels. Only then would I be able to "keep the monster in the closet," as my doctor described it. She told me that it would never be gone, that it would always be waiting until the day I stopped taking care of myself.

The signs and symptoms of type 2 diabetes are as follows:

1. *Increased hunger.* This is because your body has become insulin resistant so your body cells cannot use the sugar in your blood for energy. This causes your body cells to search for sustenance.

2. *High blood sugar levels.* Sugar can no longer be used efficiently by your body cells, so it builds up in your blood.

3. *Fatigue.* You become tired because you can no longer use sugar efficiently for energy.

4. *Frequent urination.* You will urinate more frequently because there is more sugar in your blood, which in turn draws water from your body cells into your circulation to dilute it.

5. *Increased thirst.* Eventually the water is brought to the kidneys and excreted, which in turn causes increased thirst because you are urinating more.

6. *Slower healing time*. Your resistance is lower, and a high sugar environment provides a nice, comfy home for some types of bacteria to thrive in.

7. *Weight loss.* The calories that you are eating cannot be used by your body cells because of ineffective insulin or insulin resistance. The excess sugar stays in your blood and eventually overflows into the urine and is excreted by the body. The presence of sugar in the urine is one of the tests for the presence of diabetes. Since your body is not getting energy from what you are eating, it begins to break down muscle and fat stores. This leads to rapid weight loss. (9)

Receiving this diagnosis was further evidence to me that there was something else going on besides type 2 diabetes. I wasn't losing weight, I wasn't thirsty, I didn't urinate frequently, and my healing was normal. The reasons that I was diagnosed with type 2 diabetes were that I was overweight, I was over forty, I was under stress, and my A1C blood glucose tests were elevated into the diabetic range.

The benefit of this whole episode was that it prompted me to keep track of my information: blood glucose levels, AM and PM weights, diet, exercise levels, and overall well-being.

CHAPTER SEVEN

Your Experiment

I think I have made the case that we are all different. We may have qualities in common, but our differences not only make us unique but also give us the opportunity to evaluate our own bodies and make the decisions that are best for us. Things that may work for others do not necessarily work for everyone. To find the best way for you to lose weight, you must set up an experiment to familiarize yourself with how your body works. You now have a basic familiarity with metabolic processes, metabolism, and its extreme complexities. Do not let this be daunting; you do not have to understand everything about it. In fact no one does; research is ongoing. We accept that everyone will function just a little differently, which can make a huge difference.

The following is a list of things to track. Some may seem unnecessary, but begin by tracking everything you can, and personalize it by adding some of your own categories. Then gradually eliminate the categories that you find are not helping your self-evaluation efforts. You do not want to be a few months into this effort just to find out that you should have been considering additional information.

1. **Weight.**—Track your weight every day at the same time. I do it once in the morning and once at night. It is very important to have an accurate, dependable scale. Keep everything the same, including what you wear at the weigh in. Urinate immediately before you weigh, remove jewelry, and remember that wet hair is heavy if you weigh after your shower. Just be aware of what will influence the accuracy of your weigh in, such as alcohol intake, fiber intake, salt intake, bowel movements, etc.

2. **Fluid intake**. We all need fluid. We evolved with a built-in mechanism to signal us when we need to drink. Listen to your body; keep it well hydrated, but be careful not to overdo it. Our metabolic processes are really a complicated series of chemical reactions. We do not want to interfere with the balance so they cannot perform or are inefficient. Pay attention to how much fluid you need under various conditions. You should also be careful what you drink, as it can be a quick way to consume a lot of calories.

3. **Energy use**. I don't want to call this exercise—most people see this as running or lifting weights. I suggest that you just track this as activity level. Did you have an active day? Cleaning, washing, yard work, and walking your dog all count as activity. Some people track with a pedometer that measures the number of steps they take in a day. Take a look at your own life and determine your normal level of activity in a typical day. Then look at small, easy ways to add a little more activity, like parking further from the mall or wearing sneakers more often so you can walk faster. Every little addition counts.

I want to point out that I do not believe that heavy duty exercise is necessary. In fact, it may actually be counterproductive because it doesn't burn as many calories as people expect and it makes you hungry and thirsty. At least in the beginning, be careful with the intensity of your activity until you can evaluate its effect on your weight loss. I have developed my own activity scale of 1 to 5, one being very sedentary and five being one of those days when you cannot get things done fast enough.

4. **Hunger**. Was this a hungry day? Sometimes I am hungry all day long, and other days I forget to eat because I'm so busy and not even really hungry. Evaluating this will help you to control your hunger level. Take a look at what influences your hunger; it could be the type of food you consume, activity levels, or even boredom. Then devise a way to circumvent the situations that cause you to be hungry.

5. **Sunshine**. Did you get some sun today? I mean actual exposure on your skin, for about ten minutes. I have found that a little every day works better than exposure all at once for a longer time with none for the next several days. Everyone is different and has different

tolerance for the sun. You *must* discuss this with your doctor and conduct your sun exposure in the safest way possible for your skin type. Building a natural tan is your body's way of protecting you from the sun, discuss with your doctor the safest way to get a little sun exposure. Getting a burn is always bad and should be avoided. Using sunscreen can give a false sense of security, and people get overexposed because they spend a longer time in the sun while not using sunscreen correctly, either by sweating it off or not reapplying it often enough.(10)

6. **Energy levels**. How did you feel today? Was it a good day or a lazy day? Were you all bouncy and happy, or did you just sit and pet your dog all day?

7. **Bodily functions**. Is everything working as it should be—no stop-ups or aches and pains?

8. **Unusual signs.** Quickly evaluate your overall condition. Is your vision blurry? Are you dizzy or nervous? Do you have unusual black and blue spots, rashes or itchiness, dry skin, or a dry scalp? Track anything unusual and be sure to mention it to your doctor.

9. **Do your normal tracking.** If you have type 2 diabetes and track your blood sugar or any other conditions that you are aware of, note any changes that may occur. You might be pleasantly surprised; the changes might be good as you begin to fine tune your metabolism.

I have included a chart for you to customize and use to collect your personal data.

You should consult with your doctors before embarking on this journey, as they should be aware of what you're doing and may want you to track additional data. Ideally you should be sharing your data with your doctor, whose knowledge of your specific health history may enable them to offer additional ideas and suggestions for your success.

Date	Weight		Blood Glucose		Fluids	Act. Level	Energy Level	Hunger Level	Sun Exp.	Bodily Func.	Unusual Signs	Special Occ.	Attitude	Calories Pro/Carb/Fat	Feel the Burn?
	AM	PM	AM	PM	Ozs.	0-9	L/M/H	0-4	Int/Min						

CHAPTER EIGHT

Tricks and Techniques

Following are some tips that I have found helpful during dieting.

1. Put off eating. If you aren't really hungry, then don't eat. Don't eat just because it is time or others are eating; you might be hungry later. Those are just extra calories that you don't need. The best thing I ever did was put an apple in my purse. It was insurance against "the shakes." I could put off taking in needless calories until I was truly hungry, and if that happened before food was available, I was covered by my little healthy snack. As I increased my levels of MSH my body began to burn stored fat. I began to encounter "the shakes" less often. That apple was in my purse for a long time; I had to throw it away and replace it with a new one. What does that tell you?

2. Learn to tell when you are actually hungry. Are you hungrier in the morning, at noon, or before bed? Whenever it is, don't waste your calories when you aren't hungry just because other people are eating. Go for a walk, listen to music, or catch up on reading. Eat only when your body tells you that you need nourishment. Do not listen to other people's fables, like "you must always eat breakfast" or "don't eat late in the evening just before bed." Listen to your body. Learn your natural rhythm and go with it.

3. Be careful with exercise. Movement is a good thing, but keep it at a minimum until you know your limits. Don't over-exercise and possibly kick start your hunger. That would be counterproductive. Enjoy your movement, whether it is out in the sun, listening to music or with a close friend. Eventually you can kick it up to sculpting an area of your body, there is no time line, just enjoy yourself! When I walk, I bring my puppy, and she brings me joy. I think how fortunate I am, how nothing hurts, that everything works, and that I am happy. This is the place you should strive to be.

4. Keep copious notes. Do your daily weigh-in using the chart in this book, or create one specifically for you. Learn how to rank your effort levels, mood, functions, feelings, etc. Ideas for the daily charting are in chapter 7. You can keep track of your percentages of fat, protein, carbohydrates, fiber, water, caffeine, alcohol, vitamins, minerals, sunlight, stress, happiness/mood swings, medications, bowel movements, water retention, and alertness. All of these will give you an extensive amount of information when you start to look at your overall well-being and how it affects your weight and ability to diet. Nothing is worse than following a program for months, being unsuccessful and then realizing that you should have tracked and evaluated additional data.

5. Keep a daily schedule. We are creatures of habit, and our habits can be good or bad. Bad habits can be expensive, like a three-dollar coffee full of calories each day. Choose an alternative ahead of time. Know where there is a good cup of low-calorie, good-tasting joe. Have quick fixes available. I carry packets of artificial sweetener, powdered creamer, a few special tea bags, or an herbal broth packet.

6. Surround yourself with good friends that are supportive and active. Social outings should include activities like tennis, golf, dancing, bike riding, swimming, or hiking. If you have a group of friends that only meet to eat and drink, you are setting yourself up for a difficult time.

7. Don't get bored with your food. Use the Internet to search for new recipes. I never make the same thing twice. I figure there is so little time and so many spices that I will never be bored.

8. Stick with the type of food that works for you. Vary the percentages of fat, carbohydrates, and protein until you become proficient at losing weight. These percentages will be different for each person. Use your chart to record types of food and calories so you can determine what makes you successful.

9. Don't apologize for dieting. Bring what you need or order within your bounds. If your friends don't like it, get new friends. It is your health that is important; without that you have nothing—no friends, no family, and no life.

10. Donate your big clothes. As soon as you shrink out of your clothes, donate them. Keep yourself in well-fitting, good-looking clothing and never look back. Only look forward to your next goal. I make mine in short steps—five-pound intervals. The day I weighed less than my husband was a day of celebration.

11. Take time to look at how your life is changing. My big accomplishment was to be comfortable and not embarrassed in an airplane seat. I took way too much pleasure in turning down the snacks and crossing my legs comfortably. Small everyday things are so much more pleasurable, like walking, shopping for clothes in a normal store, or wearing more stylish clothing.

All of these things are great motivators. Don't bemoan what you cannot do anymore. Instead, look forward to all the great things that you can now enjoy doing.

CHAPTER NINE

What Do You Weigh?

When you get on the scale, what do you weigh? You see a number, but what are you weighing? Your total body, not just your fat. When you are dieting, it is all too common to see a change on the scale and attribute it to the amount of fat either gained or lost. Huge mistake. You are made up of many different fluids, solids, chemicals, and structures, every one of which can decrease or increase in mass. Most of us can tell when we are holding water. This is very cyclical for women and also dependent on things like the amount of salt consumed or exercise intensity. Remember, your body responds to the environment minute to minute. If you start to exercise intensely, your body is going to try to preserve water as well as make you thirsty. This means that after an intense workout, you may actually experience a weight gain. You have to take these things into account when you are evaluating your data. It may take a month to see results that you can determine by the scale. Also, muscle weighs more than fat; it uses more calories on a daily basis. This is why we are encouraged to build muscle, so at our resting rate we burn more calories.

I strongly encourage you to look at the long term trend lines when evaluating your data; a graph is going to tell you much more than day to day numbers. Also, keep this in mind when you have a good day of restricting your caloric intake only to see the scale not reward you the next day. Remember, this is a long-term lifestyle change, and it is the trend line that is important.

CHAPTER TEN

Prepare for Success

With the knowledge that you have acquired, I know you will be able to manage your weight and improve your health. The best secret to your success is confidence. You should now be confident that you have the knowledge to make decisions for yourself. You may listen to the opinions of others, but do not let them deter you from your goal. Remain focused as you work toward achieving success. I find that small steps add up to big results. For me, I broke my journey into five-pound increments, and as I passed into the next five-pound goal, I never looked back. I donated my large clothes and bought smaller ones—even just one favorite item at a time is enough to help you stay on track. Try it on every day. Watch it fit better and note how it makes you feel.

Accept compliments gracefully. I always appreciate it when people notice that I am being successful. Soon they will be asking you how you are achieving your goals. Now you can share the secrets of your success and be a role model that others look to for encouragement.

Have a safe and happy journey!

Endnotes

1. Abdel-malek, Zalfa. "Signaling Pathways for UV-induced Melanogenic Response." *researchgrantdatabase. com.* 3 March 2002. www.researchgrantdatabase. com/g/1r01es009110-01>

2. Curtis, Helen and N. Sue Barnes. *Biology.* New York: Worth Publishers, Inc., 1989. 729.

3. Curtis, Helen and N. Sue Barnes. *Biology.* New York: Worth Publishers, Inc., 1989. 726.

4. Forbes, Stacey, et al. "Integrated control of appetite and fat metabolism by the leptin-proopiomelanocortin

pathway." *Proceedings of the National Academy of Sciences of the United States of America* 98 (21 March 2001): 4233-4237 www.pnas.org/cgi/doi/10.1073/ pnas.071054298>

5. Poh-Fitzpatrick, Maureen, et al. "Erythropoietic Protoporphyria Treatment and Management." *emedicine. medscape.com.* 5 August 2010.

<emedicine.medscape.com/article/110406-treatment>

6. Holick, Michael. "Vitamin D Deficiency." *New England Journal of Medicine* 19 (July 2007): 266-281.

7. Yanagihara, Hiramoto, et al. "Ultraviolet B irradiation of the eye activates a nitric oxide-dependent hypothalamopituitary proopiomelanocortin pathway and modulates functions of alpha-melanocyte-stimulating hormone-responsive cells." *Journal of Investigative Dermatology* 21. No. 120 (September 2002): 123-127. www. nature.com/jid/journal/v120/n1/full/5601715a.html>

8. "About Metabolic Syndrome." *heart.org.* 24 August 2011. www.heart.org/heartorg/Conditions/more/metabolicsyndrome/about-metabolic-syndrome>

9. "Type 2 diabetes: Symptoms." Mayoclinic.com. 24 May 2011. www.mayoclinic.com/health/type-2-diabetes/ds00585/dsection=symptoms>

10. Autier, Phillippe, et al. "Sunscreen Use and Duration of Sun Exposure: a Double-Blind, Randomized Trial." *jnci.oxfordjournals.org.* 7(June 1999): 1304-1309.

<http:/jnci.oxfordjournals.org/content/91/15/1304.full>

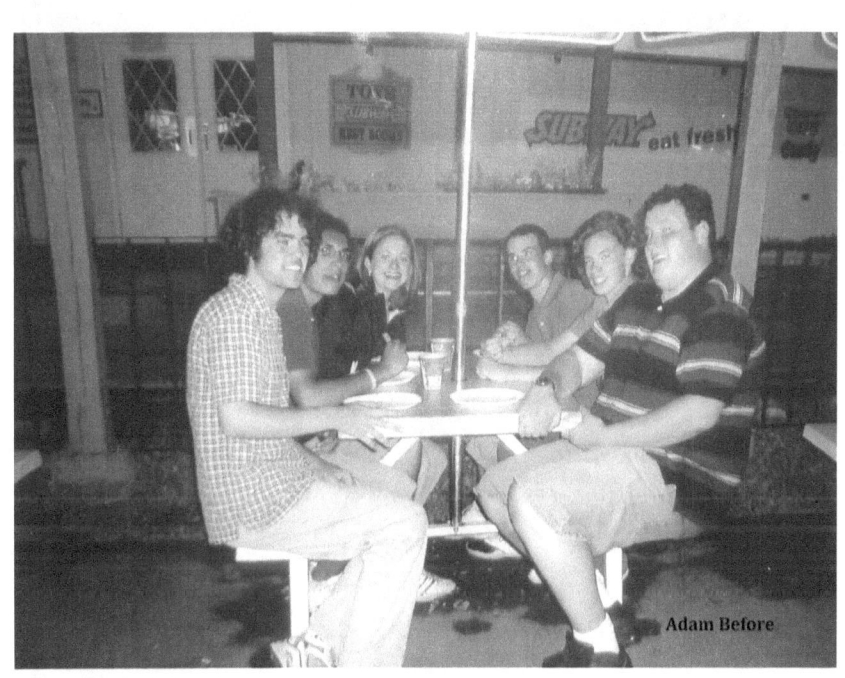

Adam Before

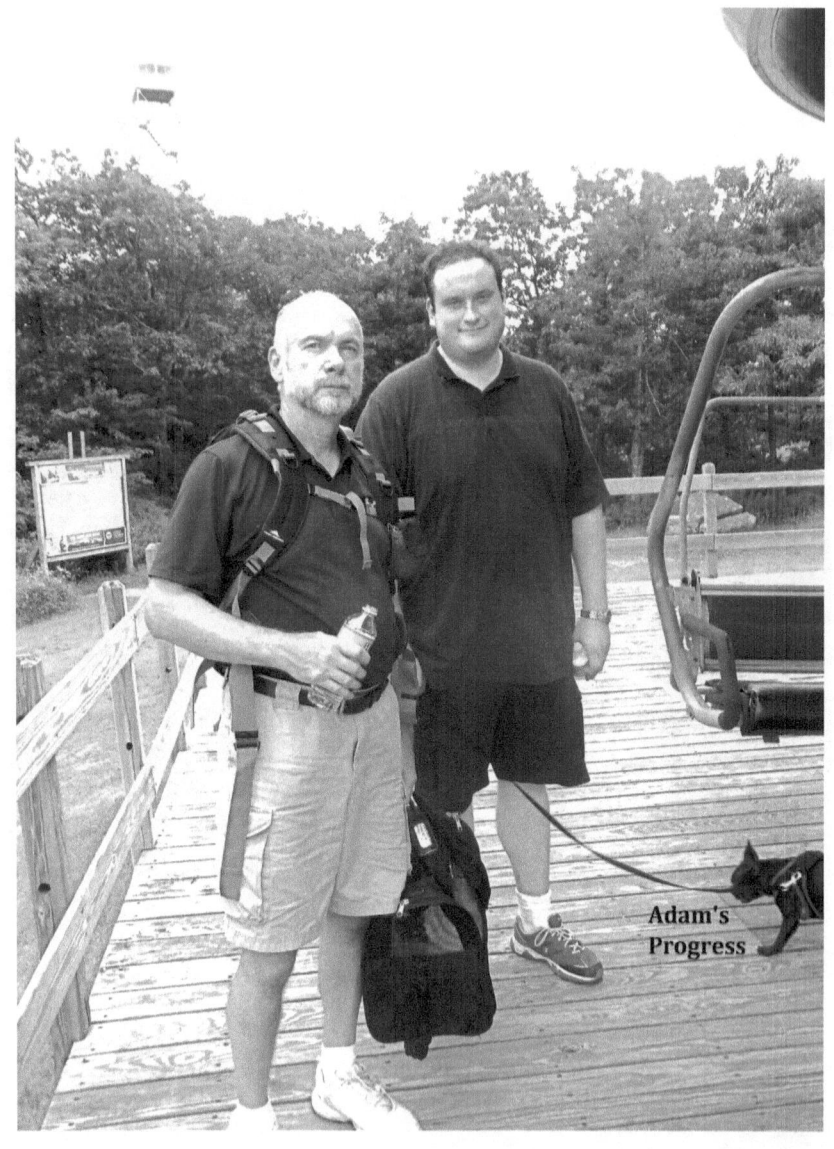

Adam's
Progress

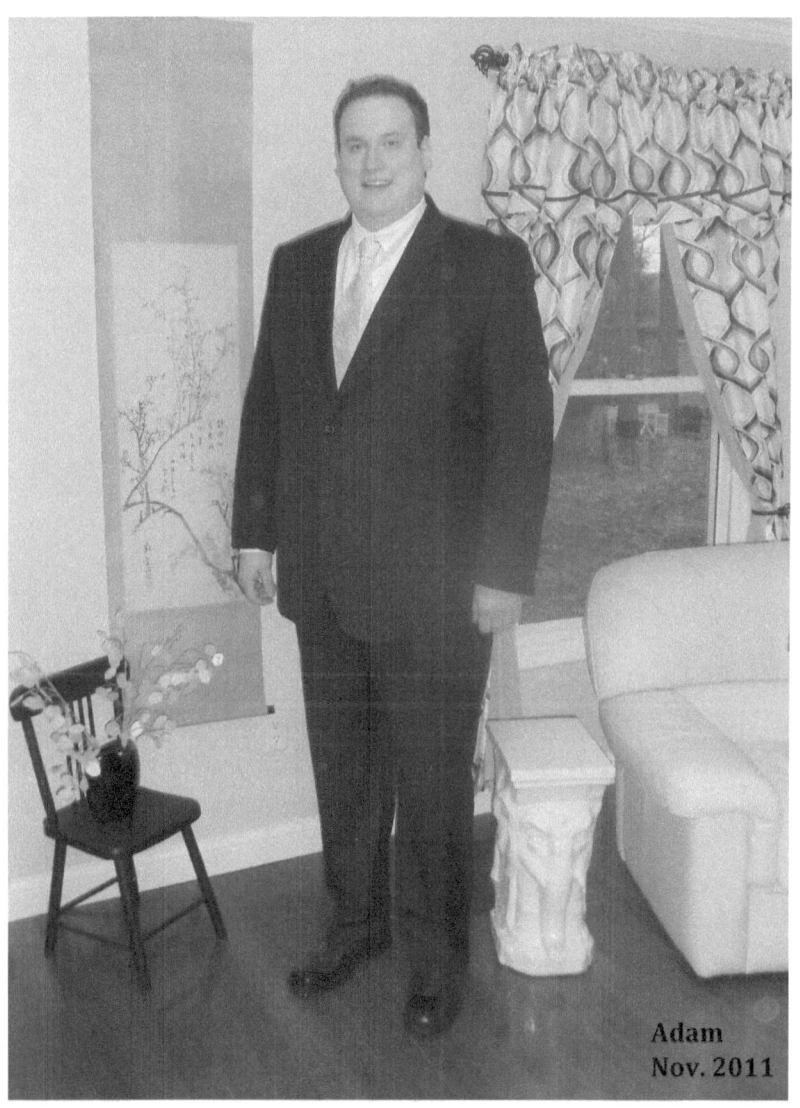

Adam
Nov. 2011

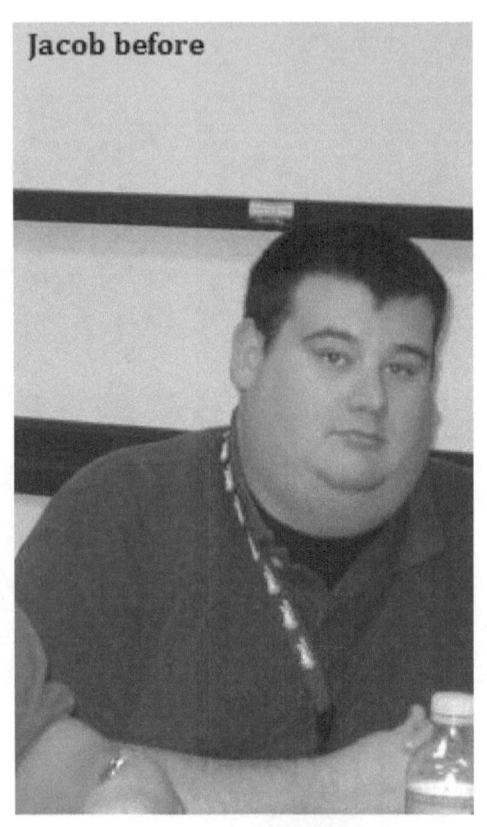

Jacob before

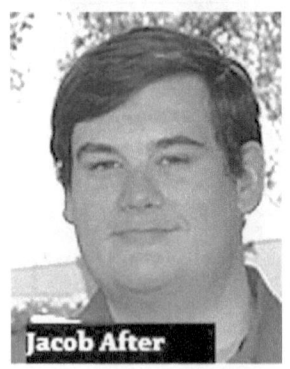

Jacob After

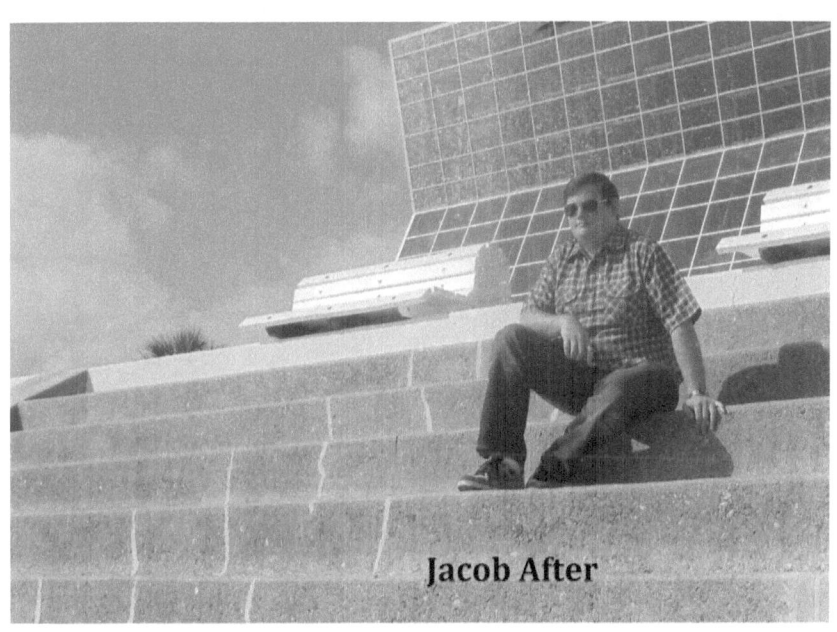

Jacob After

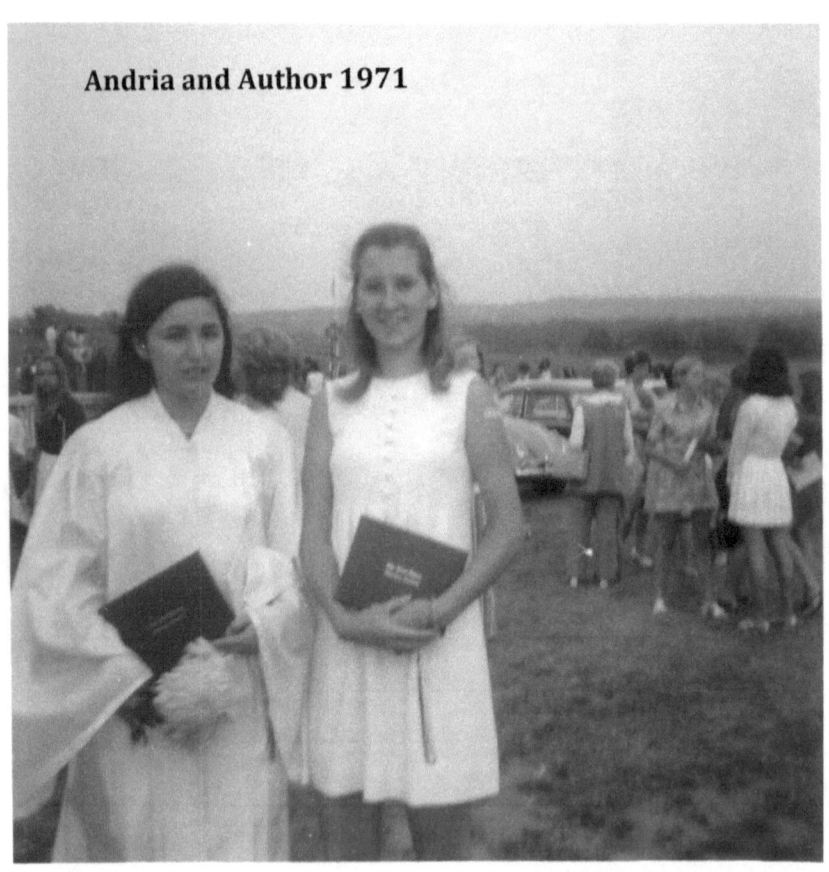

Andria and Author 1971

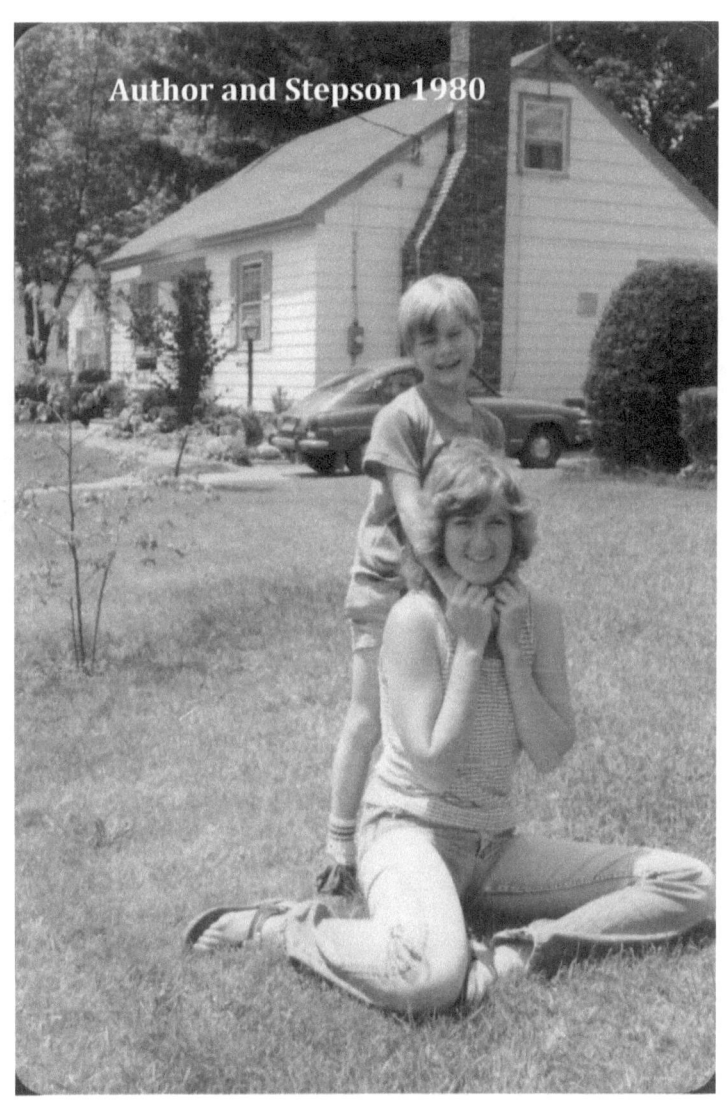

Author and Stepson 1980

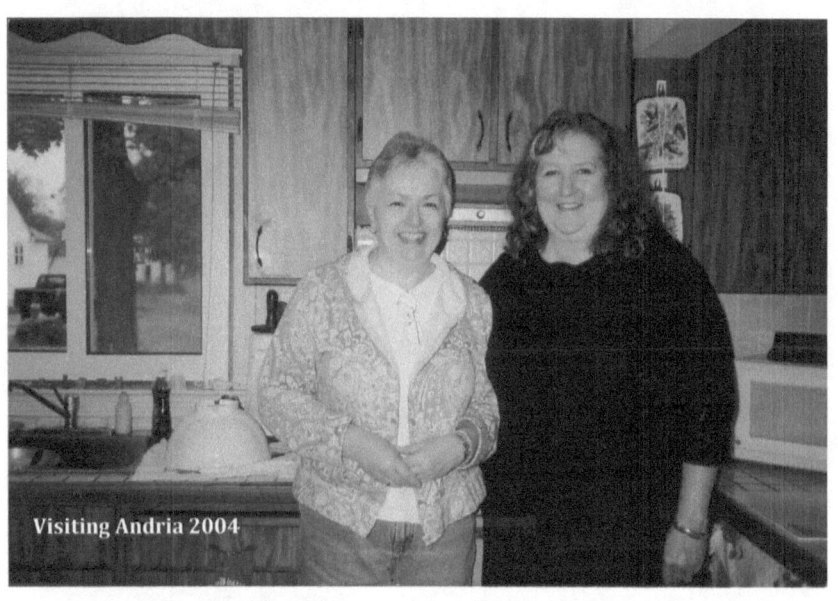

Visiting Andria 2004

www.ingramcontent.com/pod-product-compliance
Lightning Source LLC
Chambersburg PA
CBHW031242280526
45784CB00004B/1678